Nurses are The Plug

Melandy Falling-Jones NP-C
Amazon.com

Description

Whether you see nursing in your future, are a current nurse or thinking of advancing your nursing career, this book is sure to inspire you to move forward.

Illustrated by: Tori Jones, Victoria Smith, Ramiyah Wheeler and Zariyah Wheeler.

To-

God. For guiding me.

To-
My Husband Arthur Jones for unlimited love and support.

To-
My girls Kiah, Mya and Tori. For patiently waiting.

To-
Mom and Dad (Jewel and Walter Falling). Thank you for your continued support and strong faith.

To-
My siblings. Thank you for the endless support while in school.

To-
My niece, Michele Sabrina Carter. I know you will do great things.

To-
All Nurses. Thank you for your massive world contributions.

To-
Future nurses. Keep moving forward.

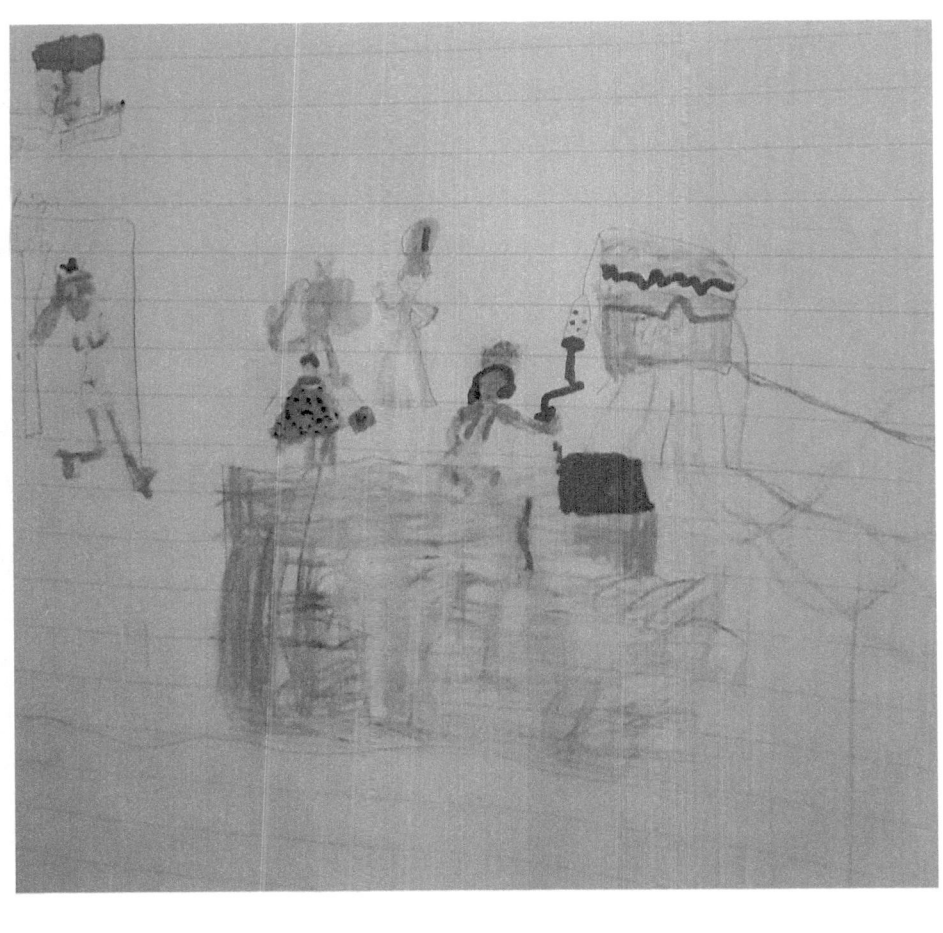

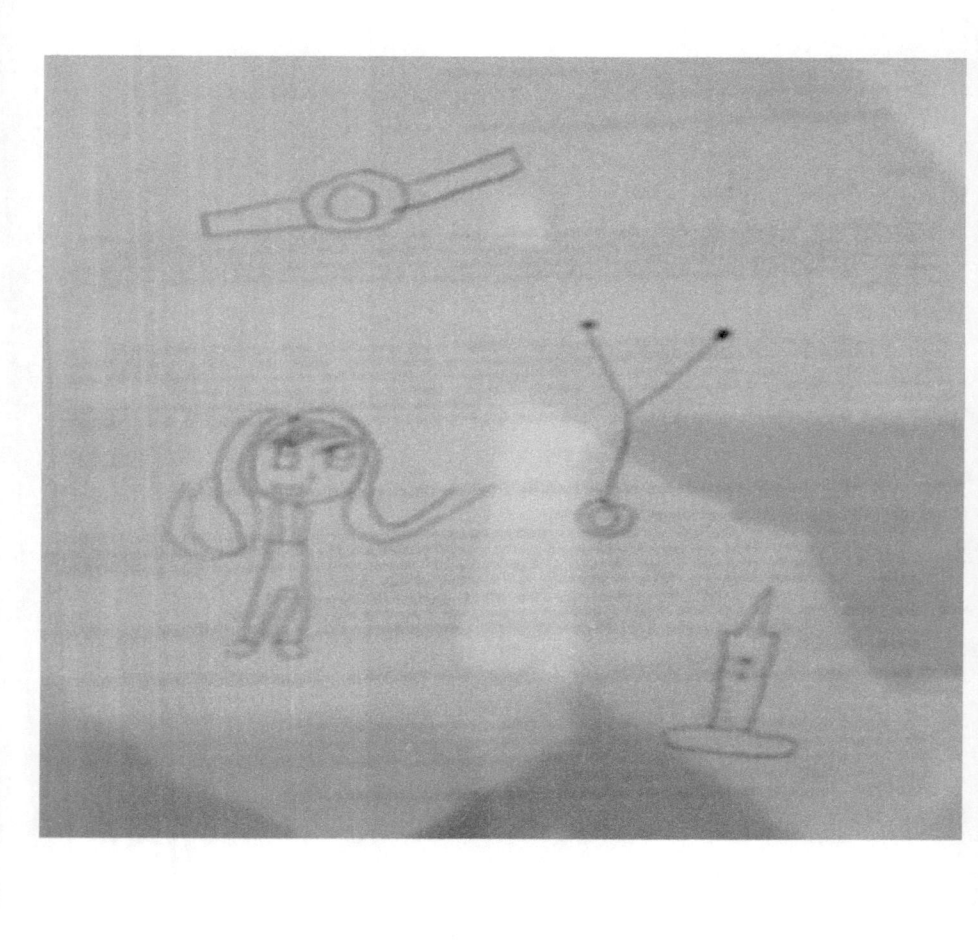

Zaniyah

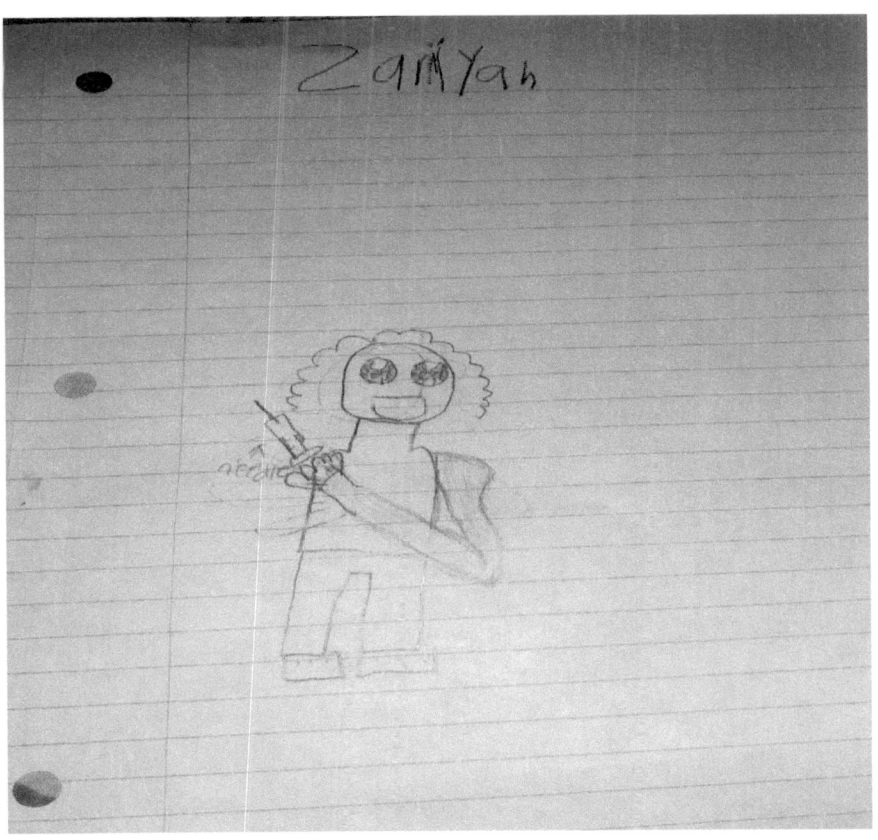

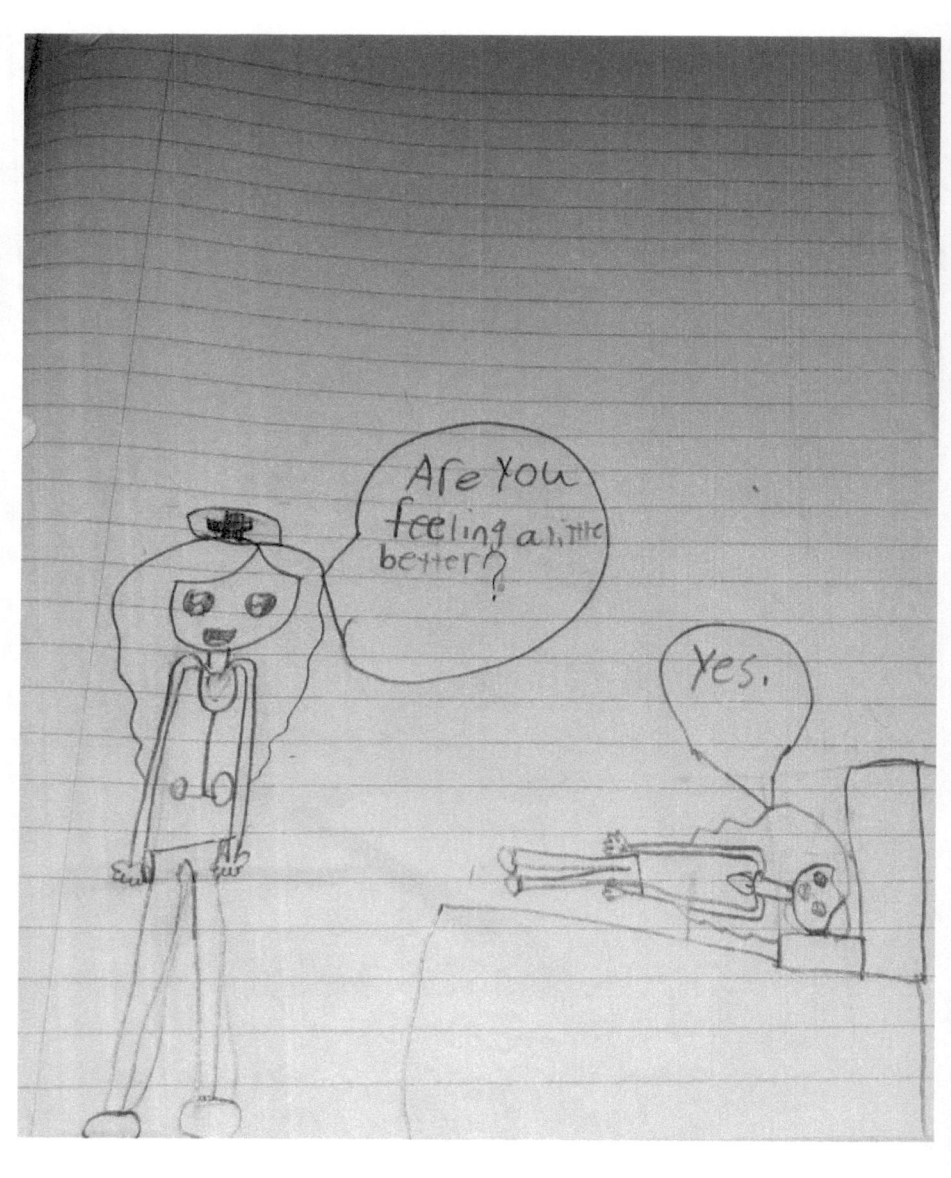

Contents

Part 1 Introduction

As a child I loved school. I watched the teachers, I collected papers, pens, pencils and loved everything about it. Once my granddad took my cousins and I to get old notebooks from a pile of disposed papers from the local pharmacies. I thought that I was in heaven. My cousins Nicole, John, Regina, Walter and Bernard watched from the back of grandad's truck as I passionately grabbed as much as I could get my hands on. I carefully snatched up every outdated receipt book, because I could use it to play school with my dolls. I showed passion and excitement when it came to playing school. I loved learning. Mom nurtured me, gave me motherly love, comforting lectures, lessons, kisses and hugs that were hard to match. Dad gave me determination. He showed me that there was always a way even when it looked like there wasn't. I've held onto that love and that determination. This same love and determination is also inside of you.

Part 2 History

There are a number of nurses that have impacted the nursing profession.

To all of the nurses before us, thank you for your contribution. Thank you for making a path for us all. Thank you for protocols and innovation. For the service you have provided. For continuous inspiration and motivation. They have paved the way as one paves the way through a jungle. They provided care, they cooked, they cleaned, they took care of the wounds. True example of holistic care.Their passion was to serve the people, their community. It is now our turn.

Hugs and love
Ask for guidance on serving holistically
You're moving the world

Part 3 Who are you doing this for?

Understand the reason for your hope. Why do you do what you do? Why do you want to do it? Will you stand firm for it? Are you stable in the reasons for you going after this degree? After this new venture? For choosing this career? Do you still feel the same after a number of years? Do you remember why you came in this direction? Don't forget why you came. Take some time to reflect on the "whys." Don't go into this for money. Do your research.

Hugs and love

Ask for guidance on clarity
Take some quiet time
You're absolute

Part 4 Who's Gonna Jump In

Everyone is a little scared initially, as with any new venture. Whether it's enrolling into nursing school or accepting a new nursing position, it all takes tremendous courage. It separates those who do, from those who don't. For those who do..... get ready. It will be a challenge. One of the greatest challenges of your life. During this challenge, you get to create new pathways. You'll go places you've never been. You will learn more about yourself than you've previously learned. You will learn a number of new things about yourself. And when it's all over, you will be forever grateful. Even those who have gone ahead of you cannot fully express what is to come. They cannot explain to you what your experience will be. It just cannot be put into words. The emotions, the feelings, the mindset, the excitement, the disappointment it's all your decision to see. It all happens when you decide. Decide.

Hugs and love
Ask for guidance on when to go for it
Listen
Pray
You're attentive

Part 5 Sacrifices

Sacrifices must be made for any journey worth making. There s a reason for the pressure. Many people enter this career field with questions of "How can I? When will I be able to? How will I?" These are common questions. The ones who figure it out, make it. Which one are you?

My parents kept my three-year old daughter throughout nursing school. Often, my sisters helped. I wanted that time with her, but I had to trade some of it for what I was aiming for. These were trusted sources. She was well taken care of. Her beautiful innocent face deserved it, and it was all well worth it.

Hugs and love
Ask for guidance on sacrifices
Pray
Look for the best
You're adaptable

Part 6 Fill Yourself First

Before you can care for others, you must care for yourself. You have to know that you're filled before you can give. When you don't take care of yourself fully, it shows. You see it. The patients see it. The lack can often make the patients feel like they're being a burden. Our job is to make them feel as comfortable as possible. But our job is impossible if we ourselves aren't as comfortable as possible. Take care of yourself. Reflect on the things that bring you joy. Things that bring a smile. Do it.

Hugs and love
Ask for guidance on filling yourself
Be there for you
Nurture yourself
You're self-compassionate

Part 7 Getting In

Have you heard that it's hard, it's tough, it's impossible? What co you believe?
Like most things in life, if this is what you desire, put forth the effort and it will come to you.
Getting into school, getting into that new position, getting into anything. You will get to where
you need to go if you put forth the desire, the persistence and consistency. Do your research.
Just don't stop.

Hugs and love

Ask for guidance on perseverance
Keep moving
Apply to more than one school
You're determined

Part 8 Knowing Your Learning Type

Everyone has a learning type that is much more suitable for them. When you find this out, you can tweak your study methods and incorporate pertinent styles to help you reach your goals. How do you learn best? What type of learner are you? How does information stick with you? Do you have to READ it (Reading/Writing)? Do you have to SEE it (Visual)? Do you have to HEAR it (Auditory)? Do you have to experience it HANDS ON (Kinesthetic)? Have you ever discovered how you learn best? Reflect on you and how you remember best. Incorporate the things that make the information stick.

READING-Written information, hand-outs, books, flashcards
VISUAL-Graphics, charts
AUDITORY-Reciting out loud, vides, audios
KINESTHETIC-Demonstrate, experience, learn by doing

You may have *more than one* learning style. For me, when studying, I used flashcards for visual repetition and videos for audio repetition.

Hugs and love
Ask for guidance on finding your learning style
Repeat
You're efficient

Part 9 Tips on Studying

Studying for school, or preparing for a job..Know your objectives. What do you need to study? What exactly are you preparing for?

Repetition is key. If you continue to do things over and over, it will become easier. Discover your learning style. Respect your learning style. Do the same things over and over. Become the expert at answering questions. Reflect on what you need to do consistently. You will succeed.

Hugs and love

Ask for guidance on preparation
Be kind and patient with you
Avoid negativity
Understand that when it's over, it's over
Move
You're prepared

Part 10 Filter Conversations

When pursuing desires, it is important to look and hope for the best. To surround yourselves with people who do the same. It is surprising to see how many anxious conversations you may find yourself a part of if you do not carefully filter your conversations. This is one of the most important things you can do to control your environment. When you control anxious conversations, you can control your perspectives and emotions to upcoming tests, assignments or work shifts.

While in nursing school, I listened to ALL conversations. I was terrified of some. I discovered that it was unnecessary. So, when I went to Nurse Practitioner school, I decided that I would avoid many conversations with peers to prevent any extra anxiety. This worked, but I also missed some things. Some things that would have helped me. There is one reason I recommend controlling conversations versus avoiding them. When I avoided the conversations in NP school, I missed out on an alternate book that was beneficial for studying as well as taking the boards certification. I finally purchased my own copy during the last 6 months of school. When I saw the information that it contained, I realized that some of the students had been using the book during previous semesters, and it had helped them tremendously. If only I had planned some conversations with my peers, I would have been aware as well. So filter, versus avoid. There is a balance in everything. Take in what you need. Disregard what you don't.

Hugs and love
Ask for guidance on filtering
Get into silence
Get into nature
You're amazing

Part 11 What Are You Becoming?

We are constantly becoming. You are becoming as you are transitioning from nursing school to a new nurse, from a new nurse to a master's and doctorate's prepared nurse, to the business owner to changing history. Pay attention to who you are becoming. You are impacting the people around you. You are impacting the world. Remember what allowed you to get through it all.

Hugs and love
Ask for guidance on becoming
Time will pass either way
Do it now
Pray
Show gratitude
You're grateful

Part 12 The Accomplishment List

You have accomplished many things in life. Now is the time to reflect on those things. This will be a part of your tool kit. Your survival tool kit. Your emergency tool kit.

Keep an accomplishment list so that you don't forget how great you already are. This kit will lift your spirits to keep you aiming high. It is so easy to forget. Keep a reminder.

Hugs and love
Ask for guidance on who you are
Be great
You're awesome

Part 13 Hold your hand

Sometimes you may look for someone to hold your hand. Sometimes that person may be there. Other times, not so much. Then what? Now would be the time to take out your notes. Your physical notes from training and your spiritual notes of what's going on within.

Hugs and love
Ask for guidance on self-evaluation
Have some me time
You're enough

Part 14 Things my Instructors said

Once when our RN class was stressing about retaining information for a test, an instructor laughed as she said "It's all there. You just don't know it. You can retrieve it." She was right!

Another instructor said, "Some will love it, some will not like it, and some will continue to go to school." She was also right.

As I was stressing about an exam while in NP school, I had a phone conversation with one of my professors. She asked me if I was stressing because of what people may think. I thought about it. I told her that I was stressing because of what I would think about myself. She quickly reminded me that there were more things happening in the world. Far worse than me failing a test. She told me to gain my confidence. She explained how she sometimes lost confidence, but had to gain it with each speech that she gave during conferences. What stood out to me was, there were far worse things happening. I was not faced with any tragedy. I was simply dealing with the scare of me possibly not passing an exam. I realized that this was not as important as I had deemed it to be. I let go. I passed, and will hold on to what's important in life.

Hugs and love
Ask for guidance on discernment
Meditate
Get into nature
You're capable

Part 15 Making Nursing Your Own

What type of impact do you want to make in this profession? How do you want to enhance the profession? Being........ here is enough. Listen to what is needed. Gravitate to what calls you. Make a game of what you're learning. Make an easier approach to those who come after you. You are a major part of evolution. You are making a huge difference.

Hugs and love
Ask for guidance on finding your way
Listen
You're a change maker

Part 16 Cheat sheet

Assessment from head to toe guideline. If this is a specialty area, include heavily detailed information on these body systems. If there are changes during the day, have a section for this. A section for new orders. A section for all doctors. A section for medication changes. A section for pharmacy name.

I made copies for each patient and filled in the pertinent info. This helped tremendously with reports and staying organized!

Hugs and love
Ask for guidance on simpler ways
Be attentive
You're a genius

Part 17 Types of Positions

When it comes to nursing, it's quite easy to find your niche. There are jobs for people who like excitement, people who like to focus on one thing at a time, people who like to multitask, those who like an adrenaline rush. Jobs for people who like to collaborate, work as a team or work independently. Jobs for those who like patients, those who like paper, those who like computers, those who like math, those who like data. Jobs for those who like to be stable, those who like mobility, those who like a combination of both. Those who like politics, those who like insurance, those who like community. Those who like to travel to fill the gaps for nursing shortages, those who like to work from home and those who like to educate. As you can see, there are unlimited options for us all.

What I learned from positions:

Nurse extern (Student working along with RN): I was intimidated by the patient labs...by the actual meaning of them. I found the environment super exciting. I thought that I would never retain all of this information. Sometimes extremely overwhelming. However, I retained so much of this information and appreciate every preceptor that guided me along the way.

Surgical Trauma Intensive Care Unit Extern: I learned detailed assessment skills. Giving excellent patient reports. I learned organizational skills and how much fun it was to have only two patients. I learned that I had time to research, learn the details about medications as well as intricate details that I wouldn't have normally learned with four or five patients at a time..... but if a patient crashes, I better be ready!

Cardiovascular Thoracic Surgery Nurse Extern: I learned what fast pace was all about. Adrenaline rush....patients who were acutely ill. That I didn't want to be responsible for a heart patient's life. Taking out pacing wires and wound vacs, chest tubes and that having a CABG wasn't as delicate as I had once thought.

After Graduation:

Cardiovascular Unit, Registered Nurse: I came because of day shift. I never wanted cardio because it was very complicated in school. Now I was face to face with it. I took so many notes. I learned soooo much. I was overwhelmed with classes and more classes. Pacemakers, ICDs, BP meds, Inotropics, Antiarrhythmics, Cardiac troponin, Enzymes, Drips, Cardiac Diet, Pre-op, Importance of and H & P. The Nurse Educator was awesome. I learned the importance of checking for medication indications.

Electrophysiology, Registered Nurse: I always said that I would work in any area but EP. I didn't feel that I was ready for EP patients in my life. They were delicate. I had mysteriously found that this was a whole new world of patients. A population that I knew very little about. I had already felt like I didn't belong in Cardio and now EP? Absolutely not. So, I went on my quest to find any job that did not include taking care of hearts. Fast forward. I got the job in EP. I moved afraid and courageous. I fell in love with it. I fell in love with hearts and heart rhythms. Everything about hearts!

PRN Medical Surgical Floor, RN: I learned that the staff could be comforting even when the work wasn't. That the people would be there for you, and that the coffee was great!

Home health, RN: I discovered unbelievable freedom. I would visit them in their own homes, take care of their medical needs, then have personal conversations. I loved it. I became a wound vac expert. I found that I really loved heart patients, and loved to educate on anything related to the heart.

Hospice Nursing, RN: I gained so much knowledge, great conversations and delicious recipes from my patients. I learned that I was more sensitive than I thought, that I was extremely empathetic. That I attach easily and had a hard time with goodbyes. That I wanted to make everyone better. As I witnessed families saying goodbye reluctantly, I learned that you could never really prepare. I also learned to appreciate life and being as they mean the most.

Accountable Care Organization-At home Nursing position, RN: I learned that there really are all kinds of positions available. I learned that it's really up to me and in my hands.

Accountable Care Organization-Disease Management Nurse, RN: I learned that traveling for work was fun. How being adaptable was important. That anything was possible.

Independent RN Position: It's all in my hands. Where do you want to go?

Hugs and love
Ask for guidance on finding your niche
Meditate
You're passionate

Part 18 Choosing a Job

When deciding on a job, explore. Gain some experience and pay close attention to what excites you. There is a job for every body system. Do you like the brain, the lungs, the heart, the skin, the kidneys, the reproductive system, the gastrointestinal system, the feet, the bones? There are many more!

Hugs and love
Ask for guidance on choosing the right position
You're intuitive

Part 19 Interviews

When going on an interview, find out the company's mission and vision. How do you relate personally? Know your role and the requirements. Now is time to do some research on yourself. Time to reflect on how you handle situations good or bad. What your strengths and weaknesses are. The best way I have found to do this is, by reflecting on real life situations. This way, the interview will be authentic. You will really feel, connect to and believe what you are saying. There won't be too much of a need for memorizing because you've actually experienced situations that you can reflect on. Keep it professionally related if possible. Review common interview questions for your position.

I can remember going into a job interview for dialysis. I was asked, why was I leaving my current position. I answered "Because I wasn't fulfilled." She gave me this look as if fulfillment was a luxury and how dare I! I smiled and remained constant. I was honest. I couldn't change it. Her body language changed. Her tone changed. I felt a sense of liberation. She saw that I wasn't the one for the job. I saw that the job wasn't for me. Always know what you want. Go get it.

Hugs and love
Ask for guidance on preparing for interviews
Be aware of intuition
You're adequately prepared

Part 20 A Mantra, a scripture something to hold on to:
"You were chosen to make them believe in magic." (Melandy Jones)
God will let me move forward when I believe.
Decide what mantras, affirmations or scriptures will help you when needed.

Hugs and love
Ask for guidance on belief
You were chosen

Part 21 Take Training Seriously

Training should be a time to write down everything. Or at least pertinent things. You see, the staff already knows something that you are unfamiliar with. Respect their knowledge. You can categorize later. It may not even make sense. Just write it. It will make sense later.

My take on it: This was my favorite part of every new position. Training. Orientation. My favorite because I was not the primary nurse and was allowed to make mistakes, and also because this was the highlight. To me, training made the mark. When it came to training, to me this was the start of my real journey. I wrote everything down, because I knew that after training, although nurses would be around and I would have easy access, my training was done and sufficient in their eyes. Even if not in mine. This was like the final audition. The championship game. The superbowl. The world series. City shuts down. The best of the best. So, as you can see, to me, I had to take this training seriously. When I would reflect one year later, I understood something about all that I had written.

Example: I dedicated a three-ring-binder to training. I documented everything that my preceptors taught me. I documented everything at every place of employment. When I would review, I realized that it was retained for sure.

Hugs and love
Ask for guidance on Orientation
Meditate
You're aware

Part 22 Working styles of colleagues

You will notice different working styles of your colleagues. Be non-judgemental. You can learn from everyone in some way. The person who is disorganized may be excellent with medication administration. The person who is a terrible patient advocate may be immaculate at documentation. The person who is awful at starting I.V.s may be marvelous at precepting, educating and disease management. Each colleague has their own personal style going on. Be respectful of it. Take a peek in, grab what is useful for yourself and get out. Be mindful. Be helpful in return.

I've worked with a number of nurses during my career. I've worked with the most organized, to the not so organized. I was able to hold on to a snippet of each one, store it, and make my very own experience. I am grateful for each of the nurses who have precepted me.

Hugs and love
Ask for guidance on finding your own style
You're excellent

Part 23 Teamwork

There will be nurses and staff who are willing to help you. Help them when you can. Remember the end goal. A great patient outcome is the end goal. Get together, do great things. See what you accomplish together.

Hugs and love
Ask for guidance on collaborating
You're amazing

Part 24 Use Your Resources

Answers are all around. We must know what we are looking for. Become acclimated to where our answers are. Become accustomed to new conditions and environments. Learn to do the research on finding an answer. Be consistent. Be persistent. The answers will come. Take note.

I can remember being in orientation. I was depending on a preceptor to answer all of my questions. I had a lot of questions. I was tired of asking, and on this day, she was tired of answering. She said "You have to use your resources." I didn't get offended. I learned. I learned that I had exactly what she had. She had a determination to find out the answers from a number of sources if she had to. She was willing to go the extra mile. I learned to do the same. Don't stop until you get the answer. A trail will be made. Keep asking questions. Keep calling numbers. Continue to send emails. You will get it.

Hugs and love
Ask for guidance on utilizing resources
Research FAQs
Call your Board of Nursing with questions
Be prepared
You're able

Part 25 Organize

Whether you use tabs or page numbers, organization is important. Organization makes you feel good. It keeps the process flowing. Stay on track with what is happening during your day while at work. I have found it best to take notes. Anything that happens, I document it in my own personal notes. When I am relaying a message, it makes it that much easier. I hardly ever have to say "What was that thing, or I feel like I'm forgetting something." I usually say, "let me get my notes. I wrote it down." This saves my brain space. It is appreciated by my mind as well as the person I am speaking with.

Hugs and love
Ask for guidance on organization
You've got it

Part 26 Exercise and Nutrition

Take care of yourself. Take care of you to keep your energy high. Your energy needs to be high in order for you to deliver high energy. You can only give what you have. Exercise and eating well will for sure increase energy levels needed to care for you, as well as your patients. Overloading on high energy foods such as vegetables, fruit and protein will help sustain you. Incorporating cardio and resistance training at least three days a week will increase your energy.

Hugs and love
Ask for guidance on health and wellness
You're healthy

Part 27 Hobbies

Being in school or having a nursing career can be demanding. It is rather easy to lose yourself. You must remember the things that you love. It is important to keep a list of things that excite you because it is easy to forget in the midst of responsibilities. Make sure to look at it often.

Examples: Boating, hiking, road trips, working out, karaoke, skating, writing, attending special events.

Hugs and love
Ask for guidance on sustaining hobbies
You're shining

Part 28 Do Your Research

Whenever there is a question, look it up. Always do your research. Find credible sources on the web. Usually ending in .org, .net, .edu. Learning never ends. Continue to learn and improve. Remain intellectually active. If you have a question, research. If you have a thought, research. Research, research, research.

Hugs and love
Ask for guidance on finding the answers
You're dedicated

Part 29 Innovative Nurses Make Their World

These are the nurses who are willing to create, participate in or encourage things they have never even heard of. The world is constantly evolving. And so is nursing. If you are a part of this, then decide if you want to be in on the innovation. Make your world out of scratch. Find your ingredients and make what you have not yet seen. Very interesting!

Technology is off the charts. Telephonic nursing, Telehealth, and all things mobile. We are only getting better. If you want to be a part of it, do so. Look out for endless opportunities. Do your research.

Hugs and love
Ask for guidance on Innovating
Make your mark
You're a genius

Part 30 Leadership

To become a leader of people, you have to first be a leader of yourself. You have to know how to follow, know how to relate, to understand different perspectives. Leadership is not about having a title. It is about making a change, making things flow smoothly, about listening to your colleagues, about collaborating to be successful in the overall achievement. Leadership is not a selfish deal. Leadership is all inclusive. Include the team. Understand the team. Understand that the team may not understand the rest of the team. That is your job as a leader. When pursuing a leadership role, be certain. Be certain of why you are doing this. Understand what you plan to bring. Be confident in your pursuit.

Hugs and love
Ask for guidance on Leadership
You're a natural

Part 31 The Vulnerabilities

Embracing and accepting vulnerabilities makes us human. Acknowledge them and keep moving. The idea is to keep moving. Understand that you will get what you came for if only you keep moving. We are here to transcend.

About the online computer class:

During my first semester in nursing school, I took an online computer class. I put so much effort and attention on the actual nursing courses, that I neglected the computer class. I figured I didn't really need to try as hard since it was super easy. I knew I would pass. Well…..I did pass. But I didn't pass with the grade that the Nursing program recommended.

The consequences. Sitting out of Nursing school for one whole year.

What I learned. This taught me to pay close attention to class requirements. I learned to never take for granted the small things. I learned that I needed to slow down, embrace and really appreciate where I was in life.

About asking lots of questions.

After being hired into a new challenging position with much more independence, I asked a ton of questions. Questions about everything. Everything single thing. I was extremely scared of getting out of orientation and working alone. I was new. And I didn't want to miss anything.

The consequences: The staff was sometimes exhausted of my questions.

What I learned: This taught me to research outside of work, expanding my knowledge base. I learned not to depend on staff because sometimes they may not know.

About the exit exam:

During my last year of nursing school, we had an exit exam. We would have about 2-3 times to take it. I failed it the first time.

The consequences: I was studying overtime while peers were moving on.

What I learned: This taught me to let go of putting my faith in myself and my own abilities. That there would be something bigger than me. That now was the time for me to step up my faith. It worked.

About frequently changing positions:

I noticed that I changed positions quite often. Once I learned what I needed, I would move on. It was as if I was in a flow.

The consequences: I began to feel some embarrassed for not keeping the same job for several years. Questioning..was I a failure?

What I learned: I learned that the world was changing. I heard a physician in a meeting once. He said that the new young physicians were coming in asking about vacation time. He said that the new doctors were not staying on a job long. I immediately felt my heart flutter...as if I were normal after all! I learned that I was an adventurous person. That I didn't belong to the previous position for a lifetime..that I met some great people, had some great experiences....until it was over.

Hugs and love
Ask for guidance on overcoming vu nerabilities
You got this

Part 32 The Levels

LPN: Licensed Practical Nurse. This degree can be obtained at many community colleges and are completed within 12-18 months.

RN Associates Degree: Registered Nurse two-year degree. This degree can be obtained at many colleges and universities, with major nursing courses beginning after core classes. Some LPN's choose to enter into a Bridge Program where they can obtain an RN degree within a shorter period.

RN Bachelor's Degree: Registered Nurse four-year degree. This degree can be obtained at many colleges and universities, with major nursing courses beginning after core classes.

RN Master's Degree: Registered Nurse Advanced degree. This degree can be obtained at many colleges and universities after completion of a four-year degree. Some RN's with an Associate's degree choose to enter into a Bridge Program where they can obtain a Dual degree, Bachelor's and a Master's within a shorter period.
Master's degrees may include Nurse Practitioners, Clinical Nurse Specialists, Nursing Informatics and Certified Registered Nurse Anesthetists.

RN Doctorate's Degree: Registered Nurse Advanced degree. This degree can be obtained at many colleges and universities after completion of a Master's degree.

Hugs and love
Ask for guidance on what areas to focus on
You're a success

Part 33 I Think I Want to Be a Nurse..What Next?

Decide why you want to embark on this career. Write it down so that you never forget.

Start to research accredited Colleges and Universities. This will ensure that your credits count, avoiding any problems when it's time to graduate.

If you are already enrolled in a College with a Nursing program, compile a list of questions. Visit the nursing department.

Decide if it is best for you to apply to more than one school nursing program.

Call the schools to speak with the nursing department administrator. Ask as many questions as you can think of.

Here are a few questions to get you started:

What are the prerequisites (Classes that I need prior to applying)?

How long is the program?

When is the best time to apply for the nursing program?

Can you give me information on the application process?

How can I determine if I have the correct courses to enroll?

When I decided to get into nursing, I applied to the school that I was attending as well as another school. I was placed on a waiting list at the alternate school and later accepted, then one semester later I was accepted into my current university. However, I was already transferred to another school.

Hugs and love

Ask for guidance on enrolling into nursing school

Call the board of nursing

Call the school you are interested in (Nursing Department)

Apply to program

Put yourself in the company of nurses

You're successful

Part 34 I'm a New Nurse..What next?

Get ready to learn. This is going to be exciting!

Get ready to develop a love for orientation.

Expect to learn from all nurses, new and experienced.

Pay close attention to what excites you. To what comes natural.

Keep a notebook or binder solely for orientation. Any question that you ask, write the answer in it. Anything steps that you learn, write it. Any shortcut to skills, write it. Any mnemonics, write them. Any tips and tricks, write them. You will be surprised at how much you learn as this time goes by! There will be nurses who love to educate. Listen to them. You will find very interesting and inspiring nurses all around you. Just look for them. They love what they do. They won't talk about it. They simply do it.

Take note on how you feel in the area that you choose to work. This is key in finding the area that you're passionate about. If you feel sick when it's time to go to work, don't give up. You may not like this area. You may not like the environment. You may not like the body system. You may not the hours. Whatever the reason, take note. When you pay attention to what you like and do not like, you only tailor your career to your specific needs.

When I was a new nurse, I can remember some of the nurses saying that new nurses "knew nothing." What a let down. Although I knew that I felt completely lost, I didn't need to hear it. I quickly learned that this was common for most. Most new nurses were uncomfortable, uneasy, uncertain "un" everything. After all of the learning in school, it was now time for real learning. The patients' lives would now be in my hands. And I was going to do everything I could to keep them alive! I was going to do all I could to show them love and compassion. This was one thing I was certain of. This meant I had to take good notes. I had to build up this person that I was becoming. I knew that she was inside. It was time to bring her out. I couldn't let the patients down. I couldn't let myself down. I was there to provide a service. Despite what was going on around me. Despite how others served. I had to give what I came to give.

Hugs and love

Ask for guidance on being a new nurse

Surround yourself with those who love to teach

You're excelling

Part 35 I'm an Experienced Nurse...What next?

Stretch! Try new challenges. Think outside the norm. Keep it fresh. Learning goes on forever. Challenge yourself. If you get bored, it's okay to go to new areas. We are constantly evolving. Don't become stagnant. If you love what you do and this does it for you, stay there. If you get that euphoric feel, keep it.

After hospital staff nursing on a cardiovascular floor, I moved to an electrophysiology office, rounded in local hospitals, tried home health, experienced hospice nursing, moved onto accountable care organizations where there was a "hands off patients" rule, telephonic disease management nursing where I educated on chronic diseases. I enjoyed it all. All areas played a major part of my development.

Hugs and love
Ask for guidance on your career path
Surround yourself around interesting areas
Consider advanced practice
You're growing

Part 36 I'm an Advance Practice Nurse...What next?
Think about what challenges you have not yet explored, but are interested in.
Think about what body systems thrill you, try it in this new different role.

When I decided to embark on this journey, I was walking into the unknown. I didn't know where I was going. All I knew was that I was being transferred (Falling, M., Jones, M. 2020). I followed the feeling of continuing my education. I knew for certain that I could compete on a higher level. I had a new mindset. A much bigger goal (Falling, M., Jones, M. 2020).

Hugs and love
Ask for guidance on where to go
Listen
You're well prepared

Part 37 I'm a Retired Nurse..What next?

Decide if you are ready to put nursing aside, or keep going just a little more. If you want to keep going, try something that is stimulating but not overwhelming. You can continue to find purpose. There is meaning. After all, nursing is not just a career. It's a lifestyle. An awesome one at that. Examples to consider are completing assessments for wellness visits, creating care plans for insurance companies or disease management programs. Triaging. Community services. Educating upcoming nurses. Work in immunization/flu clinics. At home nurse positions. Participating in health fairs. Volunteer services for the community. Mentoring upcoming nurses. These are all examples of positions that are all needed. We will be nurses forever. We will be asked our opinions as nurses forever. This is a part of us forever.

I knew this one nurse who retired. I realized that this was her passion after she desired to go back after an illness. She was missing it. Nursing was her life. There must be a balance. Take care of yourself. Give of yourself. You may still have more to give long after your retirement. This does not mean stress or overwork yourself Just a simple balance so that you're still thriving while in retirement.

Hugs and love
Ask for guidance on life after retirement
Listen
You're needed

Part 38 Family Life

Nursing school and careers are definitely a sacrifice. Ensure that your parents, spouse, and kids understand as best they can. They will not understand the depths of it until you are actually in it. You will not understand it until you feel it. When you want to spend time, but you're tied to a book or documenting.

Hugs and love
Ask for guidance on Family life balance
Be attentive as much as possible
You're on the right track

Part 39 Things to Remember

This world is a classroom. Life is the school.

The issues that we encounter are ife lessons...also known as classes. Classes can be titled Play more, Let Go, Adaptability, Family _ife, Stretch and so on. These classes are here to teach us how to be better in a particular subject. The class continues to show up until we get it right. Sometimes the same class can present itself year after year. The idea is to get it right. So, get it right. This is a personal journey. Go on it personally. Impress yourself.

Sometimes people are in the same life class. They can provide scme insight.

We may be in some of the same life classes right now..we came for the lessons that we came for..and we get them when we stay focused on what we came for. So...What classes are you taking?

If I could go back, I wouldn't be so scared. I would know that I am right where I need to be and that it's always okay. We are all scared. Who's going to be the leader of the scared team (Jones, M. 2019).

Hugs and love

Ask for guidance on the lessons I should be learning
Meditate
Get into nature
You're doing great

Part 40 Balance

Not too little of anything. Not too much of anything. I like to imagine a seesaw. When it's balanced, it's perfect. When it's not, continue to strive for balance. Keep an inventory on your family, mental health, physical health, home, career and education, friends, spiritual health and finances (Jones, 2019).

Hugs and love
Ask for guidance on balance
Express gratitude
You're balanced

Part 41 Goals

It is important to set goals. Aim high. Review them to see your progress. We have a path to them, but sometimes we run into a dead-end (Jones, 2019). Keep moving.

When I was setting goals, I discovered that my daughter would be in kindergarten when I completed nursing school. This could be done. This was the goal. Finish before she completes kindergarten. It gave me something to strive for. It worked.

Hugs and love
Ask for guidance on setting goals
You got it

Part 42 What do you Believe?

You are here now. Shine now. The spotlight is on you right now. Let's see what you got. Have a belief in yourself. Understand that you can accomplish anything.

Understanding that I am here right now, helped me to move and act right now. No time to waste. It's time to move. I put my belief in God. I knew that something bigger was moving me towards what I needed to do in this world. Find out what's important to you.

Hugs and love
Ask for guidance on belief
You're enlightened

Part 43 Give What You Put Into Yourself

When you fill yourself with greatness, you have greatness to give out. You can only give what you have downloaded into yourself. So, fill yourself with good th'ngs. Good moods, good senses, smells, tastes, touches, etcetera.

Hugs and love
Ask for guidance on receiving great things
Monitor your environment
You're present

References

Falling, M., Jones, M. (2020). *From Shepherds to Shadows.*
Jones, M. (2019). *I Give myself a Thousand likes.*
Find them on Amazon.com

Melandy Falling-Jones is a Board-Certified Family Nurse Practitioner. She is the author of the inspirational "I give myself a thousand likes" the children's reading comprehension book "And then there was POW!" the men's inspired "33 Days of a Rare Catharsis" and the co-author of the inspirational "From Shepherds to Shadows."